# Kratom:

## *101 Things You Need To Know About Kratom*

**Frank Coles**

professional advice. The content within this book has been derived from various sources. Please consult a licensed professional before attempting any techniques outlined in this book.

By reading this document, the reader agrees that under no circumstances are is the author responsible for any losses, direct or indirect, which are incurred as a result of the use of information contained within this document, including, but not limited to, —errors, omissions, or inaccuracies.

# Table of Contents

# Introduction

Kratom is making a noticeable mark on both the drug industry and the medical field and bears a fast-growing reputation of being a natural wonder for its countless healthcare and wellness benefits.

Since the 19th century, Kratom has been valued in traditional medicine. However, the modern world of today is shrouding it with controversy and pressing debates. The contention gives rise to whether Kratom is a safe treatment for drug addiction or a dangerous banned substance.

Recently, Kratom plants and its products have attracted attention from various law enforcement authorities worldwide. However, with a lack of reported risk issues or fatal consequences directly arising from Kratom use, its legal use still prevails in some parts of the globe.

For those of you who are new to Kratom, it is a plant medicine that grows in some selected localities of the Southeast Asian regions, particularly in Thailand, Malaysia, Burma, and Indonesia. Its medicinal leaves are primarily effective treatments of pain symptoms and opiate addiction. It has also been reputed to be a great inhibitor of symptoms arising from a variety of anti-inflammatory diseases.

Kratom leaves contain compounds that create stimulating and sedative effects to users. According to users, Kratom produces a pleasant feeling lasting longer than a cup of coffee does. Users often also experience wakefulness, moderate euphoria and a sense of wellbeing.

Like any medicinal substances that modify mood, different dosages produce a range of effects. In general, a small amount of Kratom produces a feeling of mild stimulation and alertness, while a larger dose produces a feeling of sedation. Moderate usage of Kratom never appears to impair behaviors or promote tendencies towards violent acts.

As an opiate substitute, Kratom does not contain opiates of any kind. However, its compounds have the ability to bind to the same opiate receptors in the brain that are associated with numbing feelings, pain relief and sedation. It has been said that the effects of Kratom can exhibit similarity those of opium's mood and mind altering states.

Due to these diverse activities in the brain, Kratom produces an overall pleasing feeling. However, despite its effectiveness at curbing addiction to certain narcotics, users can then become addicted to Kratom itself.

Because of its possible nature to be an abusive drug, some agencies are in uproar over Kratom, even though it mostly enjoys a long history of safe use. The Food and Drug Administration in the US labeled Kratom as a probable dangerous drug due to its properties that can potentially harm humans. Currently, Kratom is illegal and regulated in certain countries like Thailand, Malaysia, Australia, Burma, and just recently, Ireland.

In this informative guidebook, I will present you with a compilation of 101 facts that you need to know about Kratom. These numbered and itemized details, broken down across eight chapters, will ultimately form your comprehensive understanding of Kratom and its uses.

So let us get right ahead, and find out everything you need to know about Kratom.

# Chapter 1:

# Kratom Knowledge: A Botanical Background

Most people have differing opinions on what the term 'drug' really means. A specific drug is often different compared to its definition in the dictionary. For instance, botanists classify most herbs as *"drugs."*

If you strictly go by the definition of the term, "drug," it is a substance or a medicine that has a physiological effect when introduced into the living body. Since it involves physiology or biological mechanisms, it relates to the manner by which a bodily part or a living organism functions. An example of which is the slowing down of your physiological reaction to anger or anxiety by making deep breaths.

With that said, we can now determine specifically the essential nature of Kratom.

## 1st *thing you need to know...*

First and foremost, Kratom is often mistaken as a drug. It is not! It is neither a synthetic substance nor a typical opiate. Instead, Kratom, per se, is an evergreen tropical plant—*"a naturally occurring plant medicine."*

## 2<sup>nd</sup> thing you need to know...

As a native plant growing predominantly in the Southeast Asian regions, it goes by its following respective ethnic names (refer to table below)

| VERNACULAR | COMMON NAME |
|---|---|
| Filipino | Mambog |
| Vietnamese | Giam |
| Indonesian | Kadamba, Lugub, Puri |
| Malaysian | Kutum, Ketum, Polapupot, Biak-biak, Biak |
| Thai | Bai Karthom, Krataum, Taum, Kratom, Ketum, Ithang, Thang, Thom, Kakuan, Katuan |

## 3<sup>rd</sup> thing you need to know...

Based on recorded history, Pieter Willem Korthals, a Dutch botanist, owns the credit for the official discovery of the Kratom plant. While working for the British East India Company, which exploited trade and commerce in the entire Oriental sphere, particularly in Southeast Asia, he described initially the Kratom plant in a publication curated by British naturalist Dr. George Darby Haviland in Sarawak, Malaysia in 1839.

In his description he highlighted that the natives of the region often used the Kratom plant as a traditional herbal medicine to relieve symptoms of diarrhea and as an effective pain relief. The plant is also known for enhancing physical endurance, libido, and extending duration of sexual intercourse.

Its common usage, however, became more popular for the treatment of opiate dependence, which was prevalent during those times. Patients consumed or chewed the Kratom leaves to produce a pleasant feeling, and thus, reduce their symptoms of withdrawals from opiate abuse.

Nowadays, processed Kratom is making waves into kava bars, festivals, and parties. Such socially vibrant places and events are where enthusiasts commonly use and/or abuse it to get a certain high.

# 4<sup>th</sup> thing you need to know...

Korthals classified Kratom in the same botanical family as coffee —Rubiaceae. He also designated the scientific name of Kratom as Mitragyna speciosa since it contains abundantly the opioid substance, mitragynine, which is the principal mood-altering compound in the plant.

# 5<sup>th</sup> thing you need to know...

The evergreen Kratom plant can grow to as tall as 80 feet (25m) and 15 feet (5m) wide. Its dark green and glossy leaves compose an average of a dozen to 17 pairs of veins.

# 6<sup>th</sup> thing you need to know...

The Kratom plant is indigenous to the Southeast Asian countries of Myanmar, Malaysia, and Thailand. It also thrives predominantly in Vietnam and Indonesia (particularly in Borneo, Bali, and its sovereign territories in New Guinea).

In the Philippines, its common sanctuaries are in the low-altitude forests in the main islands of Luzon, Visayas, and Mindanao. In the southwestern region of the Pacific Ocean, Kratom grows in some parts of Papua New Guinea, as well as in the outback locales of Australia and bush provinces of New Zealand.

## 7th thing you need to know...

The marketing of processed Kratom has not yet fully penetrated the global mainstream markets. Hence, its unregulated availability and commercial distribution usually end up in countless online shops. Kratom products can also be found in *head shops* (specialty stores selling paraphernalia used with illegal drugs).

Generally, they come in either tablet/pill or powder forms under various brands and packaged with health and vitality designs. Its business may be a new and flourishing industry, but authorities consider the commercial trading of Kratom as an underground economy due to current controversies of its legal use, which I will discuss later.

## Chemical Characteristics & Core Compound Constituents

## 8th thing you need to know...

There are over 40 chemical compounds and at least 25 alkaloids in a Kratom leaf. Alkaloids are organic compounds that are generally basic or non-acidic (*i.e., cocaine, morphine, nicotine, and quinine*). Each of these compounds is renowned for their medicinal or poisonous attributes.

Of these alkaloids, *mitragynine* (66%), *speciogynine* (6.6%-7%), and *paynanthine* (8.6%-9%) are the most abundant. Studies showed that *mitragynine* is the key alkaloid directly responsible for much of the narcotic effects of Kratom. However, the two other components have vague properties as to how they exactly affect humans. Besides, both involve extreme complexities in a sustainable economic production.

## 9th thing you need to know...

*Mitragynine* and *7-hydroxymitragynine* are the chief psychoactive compounds in a Kratom leaf. On one hand, the quantities of *mitragynine* can vary greatly with the season of the year and the geographical location of growing and cultivating the plant.

Kratom plants originating from Southeast Asia tend to have higher amounts of *mitragynine*. If grown elsewhere, they generally have lower to non-existent *mitragynine* contents.

On the other hand, *7-hydroxymitragynine* only occurs in much lesser quantities in a Kratom leaf, with a measly amount of about 2% of its total alkaloids. Nonetheless, it acts as a reliable opioid competitor and characterizes to have the most potent analgesic effect.

## 10th thing you need to know...

Another noteworthy chemical compound in Kratom leaves is *epicatechin*. It is actually the same chemical constituent found in cranberry juice, green tea, and dark chocolate.

*Epicatechin* provides a broad range of health benefits — from decreasing the risks of cancer to reducing the detrimental influences of free radicals present in the body. Additionally, it is a very powerful antioxidant, which helps to prevent blockages in the arteries and oxidations of fat cells and tissues. It is also capable of impeding the growths of harmful microorganisms such as the E. coli bacteria.

Furthermore, *epicatechin* can help to resolve issues of urinary tract infections (UTIs). It can also be beneficial for people suffering from diabetes since it can resemble properties of insulin by biological mimicry. Equally significant is its vital role in inhibiting *alpha-amylase* (a saliva enzyme responsible for breaking down starches into sugars); and therefore, helps in the reduction of blood sugar levels.

## Inherent Interactions

### 11ᵗʰ thing you need to know...

Both *mitragynine* and *7-hydroxymitragynine* compounds interact impulsively with the principal triumvirate of opioid receptors—*Mu, Delta, and Kappa*—in the human brain. Meaning to say, they cause certain effects similar to both stimulants and opioids. In particular, *mitragynine* acts as a stimulant while *7-hydroxymitragynine* acts as a sedative.

### 12ᵗʰ thing you need to know...

Therefore, these twin chemical compounds can ultimately produce a sense of euphoria, great pleasure and well-being, dreamlike states, reduced pain, and sedation. This is especially true when users consume larger dosages of Kratom.

### 13ᵗʰ thing you need to know...

Alternatively, when users take Kratom in smaller doses, they often report a heightened sense of sociability, increased energy, talkativeness, and alertness rather than sedation. Nonetheless, these essential Kratom contents can also result in uncomfortable, and sometimes, harmful side effects. Hence, the key lies in the proper administration of dosage.

# Chapter 2:
# Specific Strains

There are currently several different strains of Kratom on the market. One reason for their overabundance is the practice of Kratom producers to combine two different types, and then, branding the resulting blends into new types with fancy names.

Another explanation could be the categorization of Kratom by its region of origin (*i.e., Red Indonesian, Green Sumatra, White Bali, etc.*).

## 14th *thing you need to know...*

Fact is that only three major specific strains compose the entire classification of Kratoms—White Vein, Green Vein, and Red Vein. Obviously, the details of the form and structure of a Kratom leaf determine and distinguish these principal strains from each other.

## Clarifications in Colour Classification

Although it sounds logical to base the classification of Kratom strains from the specific color of its leaf veins, this does not always apply. Actually, it is more important to learn how each of these Kratom strains turns into their characteristic color.

## 15th thing you need to know...

The resulting strain color does not necessarily denote the original vein color. Kratom enthusiasts surmise that about 75% to 85% of the white and green strains available in the market are originally red-veined leaves.

A fine example is the Green Borneo. It is originally a red-veined leaf but dried in a specific process to attain its characteristic green color. Therefore, the original vein color is insignificant; what matters more is how farmers process the leaves after harvesting them.

## 16th thing you need to know...

 Normally, growers dry greens inside an air-conditioned space with little to no lighting at all before drying them outside for an hour. Processing the whites usually involves drying the leaves indoors without lighting. Achieving the reds comes from either fermenting the leaves or subjecting them to various types and intensities of light exposure (*i.e., lamp light, sunlight or UV light*).

## 17ᵗʰ thing you need to know...

Other crucial factors in achieving specific strain colors are the source location of the plant, soil constitution, and season. Typically, the rainy seasons produce pale or brighter leaves, which are less potent. Conversely, harvested Kratoms during the dry seasons exhibit darker leaves that have narcotic effects and are more powerful.

While most of the white and green strains originated from red-veined leaves, there actually exist white- and green-veined leaves. These leaf species are just usually rare to find.

In conclusion, the drying process of farming Kratom leaves is the key to changing the colors of the strains. Growers will only have white, green, red, and *Bentuangie* (fermented red-veined leaf).

## Watery Whites

## 18ᵗʰ thing you need to know...

**White Vein Kratom (Tang Gua):** White

Kratom is in the opposite side of red Kratom in the Kratom strain spectrum. It denotes having sufficient water volumes during its entire life cycle; thus, it has low *7-hydroxymitragynine* levels. For this reason, producers usually blend it with a green or red strain to attain potent effects of the scanty alkaloid.

**Provided Potencies:**
- Acts as a mild caffeine substitute
- Causes muscle relaxation
- Improves mental focus and attention spans
- Increases alertness, wakefulness, and creativity
- Battles social fretfulness and builds confidence
- Relieves pain and irritating feelings
- Enhances overall mood with euphoric effects

**Preferred Practitioners/Patients:**
- Heavy users of caffeine
- Sufferers of opioid withdrawals
- Individuals experiencing pain symptoms
- People undergoing stress/depression and anxiety

## Generous Greens

### *19th thing you need to know...*

**Green Vein Kratom (Yakyai):** Noted as the middle of the road strain between the white and red Kratoms, it is neither an option that is the least nor the most expensive. In brief, it is a moderate strain. It is popular for its more sophisticated flavor compared to the slightly bitter taste of red Kratom.

Green Kratom has more balanced potent effects since it contains generously equal levels of alkaloids. As such, blending green Kratoms is ideal for achieving the full effects of each combined leaf. Typically, green Kratom is a blend of both red and white Kratoms.

**Provided Potencies:**
- Possesses similar applications as white Kratoms, but with more intense effects

**Preferred Practitioners/Patients:**
- Recommended to the same white Kratom users, but with a more pleasurable experience

# Regional Reds

## *20th thing you need to know...*

**Red Vein Kratom (Kan Daeng):** Red Kratom is specifically regional, solely a Thai produce. It is the most popular and best-selling Kratom strain. Its distinctive characteristic is its ability to grow in any environmental types, be it in water or dry areas.

Essentially, red Kratoms are sedatives. Its natural effect of numbing—similar to that of morphine—to relieve pain symptoms heightens more its repute as a potent sedative rather than a stimulant.

**Provided Potencies:**
- Possesses the most potent effects attributed by both white and green Kratoms, except that it is a powerful sedative, albeit, effects of milder mood enhancements also arise from the strain.

**Preferred Practitioners/Patients:**
- Highly advisable for opiate-dependent patients since it matches most of the sensory effects of opiate with only lesser side effects

# Stimulating Strains

## *21ˢᵗ thing you need to know...*

**Maeng Da and Thai Kratoms:** Maeng Da Kratom is a genetically enhanced type of Thai Kratom. Commercially, the red and green Maeng Da Kratoms are blends containing a white strain.

Scientific evaluations reveal that the addition of the white strain makes Maeng Da the most potent stimulating strain of Kratoms. It is also ideal as a mood enhancer and pain reliever while acting as an excellent strain for revitalizing the user.

Thai Kratom is a powerful energy booster. Like Maeng Da, it has intense pain-killing properties. The white/green blend Thai Kratom is also a powerful stimulant for countering anxiety and depression. However, it is deficient with analgesic qualities.

## Sedating Strains

### 22nd *thing you need to know...*

**Indo, Bali and Borneo Kratoms:** Borneo Kratom is a stronger muscle relaxant than an Indo Kratom. It also has its own distinctive odor, which is easy to recognize. It is a versatile sedating strain, serving as a pain reliever and mood enhancer with lesser side effects.

The Bali Kratom is the most economical, mainly because of its rapid growth and larger leaf size qualities. Administering its proper dosage can be tricky since it has a very low threshold to effect wobbling. As a resolve, experts usually counter the downside by combining it with other strains.

# Chapter 3:
# Prescriptive Preparations & Ideal Ingestions

The market offers two principal processed forms of Kratom —powder, and extract—aside from the native leaf itself. Users take these common formulations in the following manners:

## Leaf of Life

### 23rd thing you need to know...

**Fresh or Dried Leaves**: You can either smoke or chew a fresh or dried Kratom leaf.

**Smoking** – In order to smoke Kratom, you need to crush a dried Kratom leaf and roll the particles with another dried leaf. However, this method is impractical due to the substantive and unregulated dosages of the leaves that you can smoke easily.

**Chewing** – Users can cut out the fibrous and

stringy central vein of a freshly picked Kratom leaf before chewing it. After juicing it from chewing, you can swallow the chewed material and follow it up by drinking coffee, tea, or water.

Typically, you may chew one to three fresh leaves for acquiring effects of vigor and euphoria. However, since dried Kratom leaves have rough texture, you may prefer to crush them up first into powder to facilitate the ease of swallowing.

## Power Powder

### *24th thing you need to know...*

**Powdered Form:** You can make powdered Kratom easily by putting dried Kratom—either whole or crushed or coarsely ground leaves—in your coffee grinder or kitchen blender. Thereafter, process the leaves for about 5 minutes or more at high speed.

**Prepared for the Toss-N'-Wash Method –** This is the quickest, simplest, and easiest way to consume Kratom. It is also the best method to attain the effects faster.

You only have to measure your desired or recommended dose and pour it into your mouth. Swallow it up immediately with a swig of water.

Alternatively, you may prefer dividing your dose into two mouthfuls rather than doing it in a single go. The lesser Kratom powder you pour in your mouth, the easier for you to take a swig and swallow.

**Prepared as Tablet/Capsule or Pill –** Several suppliers offer powdered Kratom leaves in the forms of tablets or pills. They also sell plain, finely powdered Kratom. You can put refined Kratom into capsules. This is your ideally convenient method for avoiding the taste of Kratom, this also works best for people on the go.

However, the drawback to using this formulation is the various sizes and capacities of capsules. For instance, a size-00 capsule only contains 0.5 grams of powder. Hence, if your recommended dosage would be 5 grams, then you need to consume 10 capsules to attain the desired effect.

## 25th thing you need to know...

**Kratom Powder Blended with Water or Other Beverages:** Among the most common practices for this formulation are the following:

**Prepared as Paste –** Here is a recipe to

prepare powdered Kratom paste for drinking:

1. In a small empty drinking glass, place a single dose of powdered Kratom.

2. Pour just enough water to create a soft paste. Stir the mixture to let the powder absorb the water completely or until achieving a homogenized paste consistency.

3. By using a spoon, scoop an easy-to-swallow paste into your mouth. Take immediately a big swig with a glass of water.

4. Repeat scooping, swigging, and swallowing until you have consumed the entire dose.

NOTE: Be careful not to take too much scooped paste all at once to avoid choking accidentally on the mixture.

**Prepared as Slurry/Smoothie** – Here is recipe to prepare powdered Kratom as slurry or smoothie:

1. Add your typical dose of powdered Kratom to a glass filled with 8 ounces

of water or other beverage.

2.  Stir thoroughly until the powder is completely suspended. Take a quick swig before it has a chance to settle.

3.  Add ½-cup of water to the glass to wash and recover any particles sticking to the sides. Stir and drink.

4.  Chase away the bitter taste by sipping a fruit juice or chewing a mint-flavored gum.

**Prepared as Protein Shake** – Although most users claim to enjoy better effects ingesting Kratom mixed with protein shakes, the blend actually has more calories. Just the same, this formulation, especially made with chocolate milk, is the most pleasant and tastiest way to ingest Kratom.

Chocolate milk masks remarkably well Kratom's bitter taste. Besides, its viscosity is ideal in helping to prevent the Kratom from settling, even when stirring the mixture. However, to create a smooth milkshake without the lumps of powdered Kratom floating on top, follow this simple procedure:

1.  Put a dose of powdered Kratom into an empty glass. Pour an equal volume of chocolate milk in the glass. (Typically, use 1-cup [8-fl. oz.] of chocolate milk per dose of Kratom.)

2.  Stir thoroughly until the powdered Kratom absorbs the liquid completely or until achieving a homogenized paste consistency.

3.  Add more tablespoons of chocolate milk. Stir again to a smooth consistency free of lumps.

4.  Pour the rest of the chocolate milk. Stir again until thoroughly mixed. Drink until the glass is empty. (You can add a little chocolate milk to the glass to wash and recover any particles sticking to the sides. Stir and drink.)

NOTE: Non-dairy, chocolate-flavored almond milk is also a better alternative for chocolate milk.

**Prepared as Juice** – Kratom powder or extract can blend well with fresh juice. You can mix it up with your favorite fruits and choice of a couple of vegetables. You only need your reliable kitchen blender and you are already good to go.

For starters, take inspiration from this simple Kratom fruit and vegetable juice recipe:

Combine all the following ingredients into a blender, and process the mixture for about a minute or until thoroughly blended:

1. Kratom powder

2. One apple, roughly chopped
3. 2 carrots, roughly chopped

4. Juice of one lemon

5. A handful of kale or spinach, roughly chopped

6. Pinch of ginger powder

NOTE: You can also mix powdered Kratom with applesauce, milk, yogurt, and *kefir* (a creamy drink made of fermented cow's milk, or sometimes, goat's milk).

## Tea Treat

# 26<sup>th</sup> thing you need to know...

**Kratom Tea**: You can also brew or infuse dried Kratom leaves with hot or cold water and drink it as tea. Historically, the practice of concocting an effective Kratom tea involves combining a dose of Kratom with 8 to 10 ounces of water and allowing it to steep for about 10 minutes at high-simmer or 15 minutes at a low boil, and then straining the leaves to produce the tea.

However, I suggest making Kratom Tea using this recipe:

1. Put 2 ounces (56 grams) of dried, crushed or coarsely ground Kratom leaves into a pot. Pour 1 a liter of water and boil the mixture for about 15 minutes.

2. Pour the tea through a strainer into a bowl. Squeeze the leaves in the strainer to drain most of the liquid out. Reserve the liquid.

3. Put the strained leaves back in the pot. Pour another liter of fresh water and boil again for 15 minutes.

4. Repeat Step-2. Discard the leaves. Combine both reserved liquids by pouring

them back into the pot. Boil until reducing the volume to about 1 cup (250 mL).

NOTE: The technique of boiling down to a small volume is to allow swallowing each individual dose quickly. This recipe produces enough tea for about eight moderately strong doses, if using Kratom leaves of 'premium quality'.

However, you can boil the tea down to your desired concentration. Just be careful when nearing the end of the boiling process. When the tea begins to be syrupy, it may spatter and/or burn. You can also apply this general preparation method with larger or smaller amounts of Kratom; simply adjust the volume of water used.

Kratom tea tastes bitter, so you can sweeten it by adding honey or sugar. However, if you prefer, you can drink it quickly with one gulp and chase it quickly with your choice of drink.

You can store Kratom tea safely in the refrigerator for about a week or more. You can even store it for several months, for as long as you add about 10% alcohol to preserve it. That is adding one part of 80-proof liquor (*i.e., rum or vodka*) to three parts of Kratom tea.

When refrigerating Kratom tea, some of its components may settle at the bottom of the container. The sediments formed actually contain active Kratom alkaloids so you should dissolve it again before drinking by warming it up and stirring it.

## Exhilarating Extract

### 27<sup>th</sup> thing you need to know...

**Kratom Syrup or Resin Extract:** You can prepare syrup for preparing Kratom tea. You only need to boil the tea further and obtain its syrupy substance.

You can always store this syrup in your refrigerator for later use. The common usage of Kratom syrup is for smoking it in a pipe, similar to the procedure of smoking opium.

If you would evaporate the water from the Kratom Tea completely, you will achieve small pellets of resin-like extracts. This can later be prepared as a liquid dose or as a sweetened Kratom ball. Some people chose to swallow the pellet directly or dissolve it in hot water, and drink it as tea.

# 28<sup>th</sup> thing you need to know...

**Kratom Food Recipe Mix:** The taste of the Kratom extract and powder can be quite challenging to your taste buds. You can use Kratom in certain food recipes. One of my favorites is the Oatmeal Kratom. Follow the recipe below for preparation:

1. Put 5 to 7 grams of Kratom powder in a bowl. Add a cup of dry or instant oats.

2. Pour heated water or milk into the mixture. Stir thoroughly for 3 to 5 minutes or until fully cooking the oatmeal.

3. Add honey, brown sugar, or stevia extract to sweeten. For an enhanced texture, add some nuts or blueberries.

# Chapter 4:

# Pharmacological Properties

The extensive medicinal properties of Kratom are still continuously undergoing further studies and development.

However, what we can be certain of, as described in Chapter 2, is that Kratom has evolved into wider varieties of strains due to its varying farming processes or breeding techniques, as well as its geographical growth origins.

As a result, each of these strains can broadly differ in its pharmacological effects —categorized principally into moderate, sedating, and stimulating.

## 29th thing you need to know...

Similar to all psychoactive agents, differing dosages can produce a range of effects. The moderate use of Kratom appears to neither promote violent tendencies nor impair motor control. Small dosages of Kratom create feelings of alertness and mild stimulation, while larger doses result in sedated feelings.

## Strong Sensory Stimulant & Soothing Sedative States

### *30ᵗʰ thing you need to know...*

According to Kratom connoisseurs, red Kratoms are more sedating; whereas, green and white Kratoms are the more stimulating strains.

### *31ˢᵗ thing you need to know...*

**Stimulant State:** At this dosage level, Kratom differs from other stimulants of the central nervous system (CNS) like amphetamine drugs, caffeine, and cocoa. It is more inclined to influence the cognitive rather than physical aspects, as follows:

- Heightens alertness and consciousness
- Boosts physical, as well as sexual energies
- Motivates the will to get things done
- Improves abilities of monotonous performances
- Raises positive mood levels
- Staves off stress, depression, and anxiety

- Increases confidence and sociability levels

## 32<sup>nd</sup> *thing you need to know...*

**Sedative State:** At this dosage level, Kratom induces your body to feel euphoric states while enhances its analgesic qualities:

- Reduces sensitivity to emotional or physical pain
- Triggers dispositions of tranquility and relaxation
- Induces overall feelings of comfort and pleasure
- Introduces an enjoyable daydream like state
- Enhances the appreciation levels for music

This dosage can also have side effects, which include:

- Profuse sweating or itching
- Smaller or constricted eye pupils
- Nauseated feelings, but it could subside quickly when you lie down and relax

# Definitive Doses

## 33<sup>rd</sup> *thing you need to know...*

The appropriate quantities of Kratom that you should be purchasing must be in accordance with the frequency of your intended usage. However, it is highly advisable not to use Kratom daily.

At the earliest instance, it is always better to stay on the side of caution than to commit mistakes or take the risks with incorrect dosage, especially if you are a beginner.

Image below will show you a general guide of the potency comparisons of the most common Kratom strains available in the market:

| Kratom Strain | Energy Potency, % | Sedative Potency, % | Pain Relief Potency, % |
|---|---|---|---|
| Red Maeng Da | 20 | 75 | 90 |
| Red Sumatra | 30 | 70 | 75 |
| Red Indonesian | 35 | 60 | 65 |
| Red Vein Thai | 50 | 45 | 55 |
| Green Horned Leaf | 85 | 5 | 50 |
| Green Maeng Da | 90 | 10 | 60 |
| Green Sumatra | 65 | 30 | 50 |
| Green Indonesian | 60 | 40 | 35 |
| Green Vein Thai | 60 | 35 | 35 |
| White Horned Leaf | 85 | 20 | 20 |
| White Maeng Da | 40 | 75 | 45 |
| White Sumatra | 65 | 40 | 45 |
| White Bali | 65 | 25 | 30 |
| White Vein Thai | 70 | 30 | 30 |

## 34th thing you need to know...

A safe usage guideline would be using Kratom

not more than once or twice per week. Much preferably, never take it more than once or twice in a month, but I suggest you seek a professional opinion of a doctor or a medical professional before ingesting or self-prescribing.

The side effects of ingesting Kratom too often can lead you to develop strong dependencies on Kratom. Moreover, you would only be inclined to swap out effectively one addiction for another, especially if you use Kratom in averting withdrawal symptoms from narcotics such as heroin.

In short, reserve using Kratom as a special, yet, occasional treat. Infrequent usage of Kratom will assure you to receive more pleasure while avoiding addiction or the development of an increased tolerance.

## 35$^{th}$ thing you need to know...

For your proper guidance, refer to Tables-3 and 4 for the recommended oral dosages typical of the current Kratom varieties.

# Table 3

| STRAIN | EFFECT | DOSAGE |
|--------|--------|--------|
| Bali | Euphoric, most classic opiate-like | ½ - 3 teaspoons |
| Maeng Da | Energizing, stimulating, pain-killing | ½ - 3 teaspoons |
| Red Vein Thai | Similar to Bali | ½ - 3 teaspoons |
| Red Vein Bali | Sedating, opiate-like | ½ - 3 teaspoons |
| Green Vein Bali | Stimulating, pain-killing | ½ - 3 teaspoons |
| White Vein Bali | More euphoric | ½ - 3 teaspoons |
| White Vein Thai | Euphoric, stimulating | ½ - 3 teaspoons |
| Super Indo | Similar to Bali, but less euphoric | ½ - 3 teaspoons |
| Super Green Malaysian | Stimulating and less euphoric | ½ - 3 teaspoons |
| Ultra-Enhanced Indo | Most euphoric and reduces social anxiety | 1g or less if mixed with powdered leaf |

| | | |
|---|---|---|
| Ultra-Enhanced Maeng Da | Powerfully stimulating and pain-killing | 1g or less if mixed with powdered leaf |
| Thai Essence | Similar to Maeng Da kick | 1g or less if mixed with powdered leaf |
| Full Spectrum Tincture (FST) | Ulta-Enhanced Undo in liquid form | 0.25ml or more |

*Table 4*

| PREMIUM QUALITY KRATOM | |
| --- | --- |
| INTENSITY OF EFFECTS | DOSAGE |
| Threshold | 2-4 gm |
| Mild | 3-5 gm |
| Moderate | 4-10 gm |
| Strong | 8-15 gm |
| Very Strong | 12-25 gm |
| **ULTRA POTENT KRATOM** | |
| INTENSITY OF EFFECTS | DOSAGE |
| Threshold | 1-3 gm |
| Mild | 2-4 gm |
| Moderate | 3-7 gm |
| Strong | 6-10 gm |
| Very Strong | 8-16 gm |
| **KRATOM EXTRACT** | |
| INTENSITY OF EFFECTS | DOSAGE |
| Threshold | 1 gm |
| Mild | 1-2 gm |
| Moderate | 2-4 gm |
| Strong | 3-6 gm |
| Very Strong | 5-8 gm |

## 36<sup>th</sup> *thing you need to know...*

To distinguish the classified intensity of effects
please consider:
- **Threshold** – denotes apparent, yet, subtle
effects
- **Mild** – implies typically stimulant-like effects
- **Moderate** – connotes effects can be either
sedative-euphoric-analgesic or stimulant-like
- **Strong** – describes sedative | euphoric |
analgesic effects; intensively strong for highly
sensitive users
- **Very Strong** – signifies powerful sedative |
euphoric | analgesic effects; intensively strong
for most users

## Satisfy Sensitivities & Thwart Tolerances: Proper Practices

## 37<sup>th</sup> *thing you need to know...*

Sensitivity and tolerance to Kratom will vary for
each individual user. If you are hypersensitive to
Kratom, then you may experience certain
adverse reactions like vomiting or an upset
stomach.

## 38<sup>th</sup> thing you need to know...

As recommended, you should always begin your Kratom intake with a low dose. You should also take the same advice when you are sampling with a new batch or set of Kratom.

## 39<sup>th</sup> thing you need to know...

When consuming high doses of Kratom, it is ideal to take it on an empty stomach or about 3 hours after eating. Alternatively, take it in the morning or around a couple of hours before eating.

Although you can take it with food, it results in reduced effects. In this case, your body tends to develop a tolerance that requires taking higher doses than normal to attain the desired effect.

## 40<sup>th</sup> thing you need to know...

Regardless of which powdered Kratom you buy, never chase the high, and most importantly always talk to a medical practitioner before taking any medications.

## 41<sup>st</sup> thing you need to know...

As a general dosage guide, especially for new

Kratom users, the crucial thing is to find out your recommended dose for a particular Kratom strain. The following procedures will help you discover your required Kratom dosage if you are going to self-medicate:

**Step-1:** On an empty stomach, take about 2-3 grams of Kratom powder. After 20 to 30 minutes, you will notice its effects (This step is mandatory every time you try taking a new Kratom strain.)

**Step-2:** Evaluate these effects or sensations after about 45 minutes to an hour. If you feel nothing, then increase the dosage; add about 1 to 2 grams.

**Step-3:** Reevaluate the effects after 15 minutes. If you deem it necessary to increase a bit of the dosage, then add about 0.5 to 2 grams.

**Step-4:** At this stage, you should already feel something more pleasurable! Yet, after about 4 to 5 hours, you might want to take more. Repeat Step-3 and add a little more, using the same Kratom strain, but please be very careful not to overdose, especially if you are new to trying Kratom.

# 42$^{nd}$ thing you need to know...

As a rule of thumb, especially for beginners, 3 to 5 grams of Kratom powder is enough as an introductory dosage for your brain's fresh receptors. If you weigh less than 150 lbs., then 1.5 grams will be your sufficient dosage to start out.

# 43$^{rd}$ thing you need to know...

When using Kratom irregularly, or for those who tend to rotate their consumption for different strains, the same safe dosage of 1.5 grams is advisable to start with each strain.

Tolerance, however, is temporary. A few days or weeks of abstinence can resume to normal sensitivity levels. Just the same, you ought to avoid any tolerances to Kratom before they defeat your purpose.

With that said, it is important to learn how to use Kratom efficiently and effectively without succumbing to any forms of tolerances. Aside from determining your dosage quantities, as discussed earlier, you should consider spacing and rotating your dosage to prevent acquiring a heavy tolerance.

# 44<sup>th</sup> thing you need to know...

**Kratom Dosage Spacing:** Spacing out your dosage ensures your brain receptors keep on performing with their baseline/normal reaction levels. Thus, you will have no tendencies of increasing your tolerance. Regardless of treatment issues, it is wiser to restrict Kratom use to only once per day if you have been a "heavy user." Taking it twice a month at the most would be preferable for new users.

# 45<sup>th</sup> thing you need to know...

**Kratom Strain Rotation:** Some "heavy users" found success in preventing tolerance by altering strains used each time. This ensures to vary the behaviors or reaction levels of brain receptors. As such, the brain treats each subjected strain as a new element to process.

For instance, avoid using permanently a single strain, say, a Red vein Thai; instead, switch to a Green vein Bali as an alternate for your subsequent use. Ideally, you need to have at least four varieties of strains to use in rotating order.

Aside from stopping to build tolerance, strain rotation reduces the possibilities of experiencing *'strain-burnout.'* This is a detrimental condition where you become almost immune to any of the effects of a specific Kratom strain.

## Efficacious Effectivity

### 46<sup>th</sup> thing you need to know...

Whenever you ingest any variety of Kratom, it typically takes you from 20 to 40 minutes to experience the onrush of any sensations related to what you have consumed. As soon as you sense these feelings, the effects will last for between 3 to 6 hours.

### 47<sup>th</sup> thing you need to know...

When taking Kratom on an empty stomach, you will feel the onset of the effects 30 to 40 minutes after ingestion. When ingesting Kratom on a full stomach, effects usually begin 60-90 minutes after ingestion.

### 48<sup>th</sup> thing you need to know...

When taken in either gelatin or vegetarian capsules, the effects are much delayed than usual since it takes more time for the capsules to dissolve in your stomach.

## 49th thing you need to know...

In general, effects of white Kratom last for about 3 hours; red Kratom for roughly 5 hours; and, green Kratom can last for as long as 8 hours.

## 50th thing you need to know...

However, effectivity of the Kratom ingested depends on how accustomed you are to the effects of each Kratom strain. If you have developed tolerances to the different strains, you will most likely feel much less of an impact than you would have when first taking the supplement.

## Current Costs

## 51st thing you need to know...

A crucial point to note in the pricing of Kratom depends on quantity, quality, and the type of Kratom. Foremost, the prices of Kratom capsules are much different from plain powder, extracts, leaves, resins, or tinctures. Although loose powders and the contents of the capsule are almost similar, capsules are costlier since you can take them conveniently in pill form.

## 52$^{nd}$ thing you need to know...

The prevailing price of Kratom powder ranges from $12 to $21 per ounce.

Capsulated Kratoms cost an average of $16 per 1-ounce bottle.

Kratom resins cost around $15 per 15 grams (this means it takes 15 grams of Kratom leaves to make pure Kratom resin).

Kratom tinctures or concentrates go for as low as $100 per 6ml bottle to as high as $430 per 30ml bottle.

Kratom extracts are more expensive than the classical Kratom powder because they are super-concentrated preparations. The upside to taking it is in smaller doses to attain desired effects. Generally, the full dose ranges between 0.5 gm and 1 gram. Meaning, its ultimate price turns out the same as those powders per dose.

## 53$^{rd}$ thing you need to know...

In comparison to most medical drugs, Kratom is much less expensive. This price advantage derives from the fact that you only need to take smaller doses of Kratom to feel the effects instantly. Unlike other medical drugs, your doctor addresses your health issue with several medicines for you to buy and take them within a definite duration, which often stretches for weeks. In the end, these prescribed medical drugs can really hurt your pocket!

## 54<sup>th</sup> *thing you need to know...*

Therefore, when you look for Kratom products at their best prices and receive the ultimate value for your money, common sense dictates that you ought to compare the price with the quality of the product. In addition, since the marketing of Kratom exists predominantly in online shops, you should know the reliability and trustworthiness of these sources.

Finding ways to buy and use Kratom effectively can be challenging. It involves lots of trial and error; so, when purchasing Kratom, please ensure to do your due diligence on the trustworthiness of the company/website where you will be purchasing.

# Chapter 5:
# Bonuses & Benefits

Kratoms recent appearance on the news has attracted a lot of attention. A recent publication by CNN has detailed the beneficial impacts Kratoms have had on the lives of a multitude of people worldwide suffering from debilitating pain and those struggling with narcotics addiction, particularly opium, heroin, and amphetamine abuses. This caused quite a stir and started a debate as to the benefits and dangers of using Kratom. Let's explore those now.

## Inflammatory Illnesses Inhibitor

### *55ᵗʰ thing you need to know...*

Kratom has a diversity of medicinal effects due to its unique profile of organic compounds. As a versatile herbal medicine, it serves as a strong agent for inhibiting a variety of illnesses largely attributed to inflammation:

- Anticonvulsant (relaxes the muscles)

- Antidepressant (alleviates depression)
- Antidiarrheal (treats diarrhea)
- Anti-inflammatory (reduces inflammation)
- Antileukemic (acts against leukemia)
- Antimalarial (prevents malaria)
- Antipyretic (relieves fever)
- Antitussive (suppresses a cough)
- Anxiolytic (reduces anxiety)
- Boosts energy levels
- Lifts up moods to euphoric heights
- Stimulates immune system
- Lowers hypertension and blood sugar levels
- Nootropic (enhances cognitive functions)
- Opiate maintenance (as a substitute substance)
- Opiate withdrawal relief
- Pain relief

## Traditional Therapies & Treatments

### 56th thing you need to know...

Historically, early users of Kratom found its leaves as effective treatments to overcome stress. In particular, male manual laborers used Kratom to enhance their physical endurance as a means of averting the stresses of hard work.

### 57th thing you need to know...

Early wellness documents in Malaysia and

Thailand also reveal that the application of Kratom has become an affordable and popular alternative substance for using opium. Nevertheless, there have never been any substantive clinical tests and medical studies to help people understand the extensive health effects of Kratom.

Even the future expectations of Kratom assessed by both the U.S. Food and Drug Administration (FDA) and the Drug Enforcement Administration (DEA) appear to be gloomy. Yet, there has been a slew of recorded benefits for using or taking Kratom in specific forms. Some of the principal applications include:

## 58th thing you need to know...

**Therapy for Opiate Addiction:** Kratom has been increasingly popular among people suffering from opiate addiction and trying to get off the hook of illegal drugs. The compounds in the Kratom leaf help to reduce the side effects of opium withdrawal as they mimic most of the sensations and effects that opioids provide to users.

In Asia, many recovering drug addicts chew Kratom leaves that produce a consistent and psychological effect to battle the symptoms of opiate withdrawal. Additionally, compared to using harsher drugs, the method of chewing the leaves provides a safe and instant boost related to their addiction.

## 59ᵗʰ thing you need to know...

In comparison to opioid use, *respiratory depression* or slowed breathing has never been part of the effects of Kratom use. Respiratory depression is a typical and deadly factor in opioids abuse since opium has the ability to shut down the respiratory system, particularly during an overdose.

## 60ᵗʰ thing you need to know...

As confirmed by research, Kratom can have addictive qualities, only because of its pleasurable effects. Sometimes, this type of addiction is simply an interpretation of a developing tolerance for heavy and daily users. Fact is that nearly none of the plant's elements is addictive. Thus, in reality, the abuse potential of Kratom can be very low.

## 61ˢᵗ thing you need to know...

Since Kratom is an unregulated product, only a few studies about the plant are reliable.

However, many anecdotal reports support the beneficial role of Kratom in helping people to overcome opioid withdrawals.

## 62$^{nd}$ thing you need to know...

The American Association of Pharmaceutical Scientists (AAPS) confirmed that alkaloid compounds in Kratom could bond easily to opioid receptors in the body. As such, these compounds cause the release of *dopamine* and *serotonin* (chemical substances responsible for transmitting nerve impulses in certain brain cells to help control moods and emotions, as well as to regulate movement), just as opioid drugs typically do.

Kratom however releases the substance at more manageable levels compared to heroin or prescription pills. Thus, the symptoms of opium withdrawal become less severe.

## 63$^{rd}$ thing you need to know...

**Acute and Chronic Pain Reliever:** The most important and popular reason for using Kratom is the effectiveness of its opium-like qualities for alleviating pain. Pharmaceutical studies actually concluded favorable evaluations for using the rich analgesic properties of Kratom leaves in the self-treatment of chronic pains typically experienced in abrupt withdrawals of opioid abuse.

## 64ᵗʰ thing you need to know...

Kratom leaves quickly relieve pain throughout a person's body by influencing the systemic activities of hormones. When chewing the leaves, the quantities of *dopamine* and *serotonin* compounds released increases. Essentially, the Kratom alkaloids act in a morphine-like way by dulling the pain receptors all over the body.

## 65ᵗʰ thing you need to know...

**Energy Booster:** The Kratom leaf compounds virtually heighten focus and a buzzing stimulation that increase productivity levels. These inherent sensations of an energy boost experienced through using Kratom are entirely different from other stimulating substances. Kratom aficionados termed it singularly as, "Kratom high."

## 66ᵗʰ thing you need to know...

Unlike a caffeine overdose or simply consuming too much caffeine, Kratom does not tend to increase the heart rate. Such a unique quality arises from the extract's metabolic processes, which calm the nerves while increasing oxygen supply in the bloodstream for a more stable energy boost.

## 67th thing you need to know...

**Enhances the Mood and Relieves Anxiety:** For the same reason that the properties of the compounds in the plant help to boost energy and relieve pain, Kratom also helps people suffering from severe nervousness or anxiety, depression, and mood swings. The compounds in Kratom actually target to affect the brain's neurotransmitters—nerves that transmit signals for regulating emotions.

In particular, the leaf extracts augment the release of hormones throughout the body to control mood swings in more restrained ways, if not, eliminating them.

## 68th thing you need to know...

With each strain producing different effects, a new and inexperienced user may choose the wrong strain to treat their desired symptoms. For your quick guide in relieving anxiety, your best bet includes the Bali, Indo, and some varieties of red vein Kratoms. Please refer back to Image-3.

## 69<sup>th</sup> thing you need to know...

**Sexual Activity Enhancer:** Traditionally, Kratom practitioners have long branded the wonder plant as an aphrodisiac. Its botanical properties were renowned to aid in premature ejaculation, as well as increasing fertility in men.

While there have been no scientific studies showing evidence of its sexual effects, laboratory studies on animals revealed an increased production of sperm cells. Besides, the market for using Kratom for sexual enhancements has been growing steadily over the years. This market growth apparently manifests and strengthens its repute as an effective aphrodisiac.

# Chapter 6:

# Prudent & Precautionary Practices

Recently, Kratom has also gained popularity among the younger generations for its euphoric effects that provide a 'legal' high. Its status as an alternative to other stimulant and sedative type of drugs is also of equal interest.

## Misuse Measures

### *70<sup>th</sup> thing you need to know...*

Merchants sell Kratom products in a wide variety of forms. As a result, Kratom products can often vary in their respective alkaloid concentrations. Thus, always be aware and beware of certain misleading product labels and the marketing hypes. Some vendors sell bogus products by adulterating Kratom with other chemicals or herbs or misrepresenting other herbs as Kratom.

## 71st thing you need to know...

Chemical analysis on some Kratom products has revealed many forms of adulterations with other substances. In most cases, suppliers remove certain amounts of the original Kratom contents and replace them with less expensive herbs or other similar substance to cut down retailers' costs and increase profits.

## 72nd thing you need to know...

In other cases, suppliers add synthetic or designer drugs to enhance the effects further. These, deceptive products, misleadingly labeled as 'pure Kratom extracts' actually contain the synthetic drug, *O-desmethyltramadol*—a fatally potent synthetic opioid. One concoction goes by the label, *'Krypton,'* which compose Kratom leaves mixed with the drug.

## 73rd thing you need to know...

Disturbingly, products containing this drug have resulted in a long list of recorded deaths (with the first fatality accounted in Sweden). Yet, Kratom in its original form is far from dangerous and there has been no single reported case resulting in death after its use.

## 74th thing you need to know...

Other studies have also found similar deadly compounds—specifically morphine and *hydrocodone* (a semi-synthetic drug sourced from opium derivatives)—laced in other Kratom products. Since these are prime constituents of opioid compounds, their effects are somehow akin to those of Kratom.

## 75th thing you need to know...

While Kratom is a relatively safe and tremendously useful herb, it is just unfortunate that some unscrupulous merchants and reckless suppliers are acting so irresponsibly. If you are thinking of purchasing Kratom products, ensure to purchase from traders or shops that conduct routine testing prior to retailing the products sourced from suppliers.

## Critical Concerns & Conditions

Clinical studies are significant for the development and promotion of new drugs. They help to determine consistently the harmful effects and interactions with other drugs. These studies also help to recognize effective dosages that are sustainable and less dangerous.

Studies have found that alkaloids induce physical effects on humans. Kratom contains nearly as many alkaloids as hallucinogenic mushrooms and opium. Thus, it bears the powerful ability to have a potent effect on the human body.

Although some of these effects are desirable, others may be causes for great concern. This gives rise to why the necessity for extensive and further studies on Kratom is indeed urgent.

# 76th thing you need to know...

However, there have never been any in-depth studies about Kratom. Hence, there are no recorded official recommendations for its medical use up to now. Instead, the truth of the matter is that the limited information on the benefits and risks of Kratom in humans run counter to the over-sensationalized and inaccurate reports by popular media about the intricacies of Kratom use.

## 77th thing you need to know...

Due to the lack of sufficient evidence and available confirmations of its safe usage, it then becomes a careful forethought to keep Kratom off the reach of children. The same precautionary measures would be advisable for women undergoing pregnancy or lactation. For, after all, it is unknown whether Kratom could cause fetal death or birth defects.

# Safeness & Sustainability

## *78th thing you need to know…*

If you consume Kratom by itself, which is without any combination of other drugs, then your only greatest risk is falling asleep without warning. The perceived problems arise when you engage in hazardous activities while under a slight or heavy influence of Kratom. Therefore, you should use your common sense and refrain from driving a vehicle, using power tools, scaling ladders, or leaving a pot/kettle on a lit stove, operating heavy machinery, and all things alike.

## *79th thing you need to know…*

Health issues are least likely to occur in occasional users of Kratom unless, of course, users consume large quantities of Kratom daily. Like any other medicine, reactions vary in each individual. Some people might have unusual reactions to Kratom or an allergy despite using it responsibly.

Those who are heavily dependent on it will eventually develop dark facial pigmentations and an unhealthy weight loss. Worse, they incur physical withdrawal symptoms when quitting the habit abruptly. These withdrawal symptoms may include crying, diarrhea, muscle aches and jerking, irritability, and a runny nose.

## Toxicological Truths

Similar to its safe medical use, scientific research on the toxicity and adverse effects of Kratom are still also limited. We can only contend with consuming a few of the facts surfacing from trusted publications and medical reports.

## *80th thing you need to know...*

Primarily, a 2015 literary review from the International Journal of Legal Medicine considered that Kratom is minimally toxic. It concluded that the pharmacological effects of the Kratom leaves are dose-dependent. Meaning, the more a user takes them, the stronger the effect will be.

Although there were some reported cases of deaths attributed to heavy Kratom use, there was neither solid proof nor accounts provided where

Kratom solely contributed to the fatalities. A study in Thailand, however, documented cases of adverse withdrawal symptoms and Kratom poisoning among its users.

## 81st *thing you need to know...*

Most of the complaints of withdrawal symptoms and Kratom poisoning were under the influence of other prescribed substances or illicit drugs like codeine or cough syrup. During the last decade, there were nine death cases of intoxication related to the use of the deadly Kratom-based product, *Krypton*. However, the reports ascribed these fatalities to the addition of a synthetic opioid, which is the usual element blended in the product.

## Strength Sports

## 82nd *thing you need to know...*

Kratom's reach also extends to professional sports. The plant's analgesic and stimulating effects only imply that Kratom can be beneficial for enhancing performances in certain sports disciplines.

Technically, it is possible to detect Kratom alkaloids in body fluids. For the first time, in

2015, sports officials chanced upon detecting the essential element of Kratom—*mitragynine*—in four doping control samples coming from strength sports, particularly powerlifting and weightlifting.

However, since most places legalize Kratom as an herbal drug, it need not undergo normal testing. Protocols may likely change, especially when Kratom eventually becomes a regulated substance in the U. S.

# Chapter 7:

# Aftereffects Assessments

Considering all the positive effects occurring in Kratom use, it is important that we also highlight its negative effects.

One of the side effects of using Kratom is the notorious *'Kratom hangover,'* which carries similar symptoms typical to an alcoholic hangover. The following are the common assessments of the top five aftereffects of Kratom use:

## Chronic Consumers' Conditions

### 83<sup>rd</sup> *thing you need to know...*

High-dosage users generally experience irritability and anxiety due to Kratom's stimulating effects. Long-term users usually incur anorexia and abnormal weight loss, facial hyperpigmentation, and fretting, trembling, or wobbling.

Furthermore, the reported negative side effects extend to include alternating chills and sweats, constipation, dehydration, dizziness, itching, mouth and throat numbness, nausea, sedation, stomachaches, tiredness, unsteadiness, visual alterations and vomiting. For regular users, some have become vulnerable to develop tolerance, and very often, they inevitably increase their usual dosages over time. Others simply succumb to addiction.

## Addictive Aspects

In recent years, the use of Kratom expanded from Asia towards the U.S. and Europe. Since then, there have been steadily increasing reports of users becoming addicted or physically dependent on Kratom.

## *84th thing you need to know...*

 The main culprit for this possible addiction is the opioid-like analgesic effects of Kratom. Even though the euphoric effects typically tend to be less intensive than those produced by opioid drugs and opium, more and more drug users still seek to use Kratom.

## Digestive Damage & Liver Liabilities

## 85th thing you need to know...

The Journal of Medical Toxicology published a study stating Kratom use can lead to adverse side effects in the gastrointestinal tract (*i.e. upset stomach and vomiting*). It based its report on an individual who took Kratom for only 15 days without the presence of any other causative agents.

There have also been issues reported concerning liver injuries linked to Kratom ingestion. One report described the case of a young German who incurred impaired flows of bile within the liver after taking high doses of Kratom powder for just a couple of weeks.

# Psychological Problems

## 86th thing you need to know...

The physical aftereffect symptoms of Kratom use can peak to their prominent states but they eventually fade away within a week. Its psychological side effects can be just as typical, but sometimes, they can be more detrimental.

These damaging effects may include addiction, aggressive behaviors, anxiety, crying, decreased libido, delusions, episodic panic, hallucinations, intensive mood swings, lethargy, paranoia, psychotic episodes, and suppressed appetite.

## Waging Withdrawals

### 87th thing you need to know...

Some of the long-term users of Kratom may have difficulties giving up its regular use. They perceive a hard time to cope up with anorexia, bone and muscle aches, insomnia, jerky limb movements, psychosis and restlessness, which are the common withdrawal symptoms that follow upon a cessation of Kratom use. Nonetheless, while symptoms of Kratom withdrawal can be distracting and annoying, they do not exhibit debilitating pains as in the symptoms of opiate withdrawal.

### 88th thing you need to know...

Kratom withdrawal symptoms usually disappear after 1 to 3 days. Their common descriptions mostly connote to being short-lived and benign.

### 89th thing you need to know...

The upside for users amidst their Kratom dependence is that they continue to remain sound, fit, and trim. Besides having good health, they can still exercise normal functions, especially in their social interrelationships with others.

In fact, a Malaysian study showed no significant impairments in their performances of social functions and responsibilities.

# Chapter 8:
# Legalities & Liabilities

## 90th thing you need to know...

Kratom is legal in most countries like the U.S.A. Although the U.S. Food and Drug Administration (FDA) has long released an importation alert cautioning the negative aftereffects of regular Kratom use in humans, the botanical wonder still enjoys unregulated status in most states in the U.S.

## 91st thing you need to know...

Kratom is only banned in six of the US states—Wisconsin, Vermont, Tennessee, Indiana, Arkansas, and Alabama. This prohibition largely stemmed from a citation of drug officials at the U.S. Drug Enforcement Administration (DEA) that considered and included Kratom in the list of "Drugs and Chemicals of Concern."

## 92nd thing you need to know...

On the contrary, Kratom is illegal in the whole of

Australia, Bhutan, Denmark, Malaysia, Myanmar, and Thailand. In Europe, several EU-member states, like Sweden, Romania, Poland, Lithuania, and Finland, have regulated laws over the use of Kratom. Some of these states and countries even impose severe penalties for the possession or planting of Kratom.

## 93$^{rd}$ thing you need to know...

The current Kratom ban and control in Malaysia is under the Poisons Act of 1953. Those found guilty of distributing Kratom leaves or preparations illegally can be fined or be sentenced to jail for up to 4 years. The cultivation of Kratom is, however, not an offense in Malaysia.

## 94$^{th}$ thing you need to know...

In Thailand, officials reclassified the Kratom Act 2486 of 1943 to be under the Narcotic Act in 1979. This reclassification stipulated the illegal act of possession, planting, importing, and exporting of Kratom leaves. However, many Thai officials consider the reversal of the 75-year old ban on Kratom with respect to its valuable and unparalleled performances in weaning off opium addicts.

## 95<sup>th</sup> thing you need to know...

In Ireland, the government has just recently illegalized Kratom. At present, authorities categorized it as a Schedule-1 drug, which bestows Kratom with the same illegal status as heroin.

Similar to the US-DEA citation, most of the Irish politicians who passed this new law have never probably heard about Kratom or its potent alkaloids.

Laws can change; and, they do change all the time; so, please ensure that Kratom is legal in the area where you live prior to using it.

## 96<sup>th</sup> thing you need to know...

Like the DEA citation and the events leading up to the Kratom ban in Ireland, the status of Kratom continues to be uncertain.

## Social Standing

## 97<sup>th</sup> thing you need to know...

The most important thing to consider before using Kratom is whether you are educated enough on the subject to make a responsible and well-informed decision.

## 98ᵗʰ *thing you need to know...*

In South East Asia, most users feel confronting rebuke from family and friends for 'engaging wastefully' in the habit of Kratom use. However, either certain acts of discrimination or stereotyping them as drug users never existed.

## 99ᵗʰ *thing you need to know...*

In the northern regions of Malaysia, users easily rely on and turn to use Kratom for its beneficial purposes due to its affordability and accessibility. In cases where users struggle against opiate withdrawal symptoms, they usually hinder themselves approaching and enrolling in government wellness facilities that may likely expose their identities. Instead, most of them enable self- treatments, which help them to avoid facing stigma, disgrace, or public disapproval of their drug dependency.

Therefore, fears of arrests by law enforcement authorities and censure from the community have pushed Kratom use to clandestine settings. Several reports in Thailand have highlighted a more recent and covert trend of a drug concoction used among its youthful generation—

mostly, teenagers to people in their early 30s.

This latest drug concoction involves boiling Kratom leaves to serve as a primary base for a cocktail tagged as,"4 × 10." It is essentially a composition of Kratom tea, ice cubes, Coca-Cola, and cough syrup.

## Kratom's Kismet: Future Fate

The practices of Kratom use in both the opposite sides of the world have moved gradually away from their traditional Western and Eastern applications—treating an array of physical maladies and enhancing physical endurance—towards newer uses with much potential promises.

## 100th thing you need to know...

One significant potential that the Kratom plant holds is its development as a viable treatment choice for opiate dependence. Recent findings insinuate its strong viability option by the huge volumes of Kratom purchases from online sources by at least 40 million Americans struggling from opiate withdrawal and suffering from chronic pain. Since 2013, the numbers keep growing steadily and there seem to be no signs of any letdowns in the near future.

## 101ˢᵗ *thing you need to know...*

People "in the know" view Kratom as an economical alternative therapy to more expensive, yet, less effective prescription treatments for the self-management of opioid withdrawal, as well as relieving pain. These claims only merit serious and further scientific research and investigation, particularly for the benefit of developing countries... and most of all, to the multitude lurking in ignorance.

# Conclusion

Studies indicating Kratom's potential as a harm-reduction tool, most notably as a substitute for opioid addiction are still not enough to satisfy our question of whether Kratom is safe to use.

Both the scientific community and governments around the world truly need to perform extensive research and development studies about its uses and effects in order to form a precise and comprehensive understanding about Kratom. While the intriguing topic of completely banning or controlling Kratom keeps on heating up, some governments seem hell-bent to determine new laws while others simply remain hesitant to look back at the precautionary measures and side effects of taking this botanical wonder.

For some users, the negative mental health effects of Kratom—primarily withdrawal symptoms—appear to be relatively milder compared to those of opioids. For other indiscriminate users, withdrawal can be highly uncomfortable and it becomes more difficult to maintain abstinence.

Its pleasurable and euphoric effects only give rise

to its addictive qualities. The addiction is usually associated to a developing tolerance, especially for heavy or daily users. Actually, almost none of the plant's essential components are addictive. Therefore, in reality, the chances of Kratom abuse are very low.

However, among many users, Kratom enhances the mood and relieves anxieties, stress, and depression. Several users also rely on Kratom for its effective pain-relieving qualities and inhibiting properties of suppressing symptoms of various anti-inflammatory diseases.

These actual user results should urge, on one hand, medical researchers and mental health or substance use clinicians to consider resuming further investigations on the negative side effects of Kratom to humans, and for good reason! On the other hand, policy makers and regulators must conduct a sweeping review of current laws and regulations of Kratom use before arriving to faulty conclusions and decisions.

The positive effects on the health and lives of many users are as significant to consider. It can truly be life preserving for opiate abusers to use Kratom in a positive manner and along a regulated short-term duration to end fatal drug dependencies.

In ending, the key point I would like to reemphasize is to be diligent and responsible enough to do your own part. Investigate and perform your own research. Consider all factors involved, including your mental and physical conditions. Seek consultations with your physician as well prior to using Kratom.

Never hitch on the bandwagon of media and promotional hypes. Only choose reliable and trustworthy suppliers. Know how they manufacture or process and source their Kratoms.

Cheap prices can be tempting, but quality must remain paramount.

Lastly, I hope you have enjoyed reading this book and I would appreciate all your reviews.

Made in the USA
Monee, IL
12 April 2021

65458061R00049